PAPA'S BOOTS

Written by
Amanda Graves

Illustrated by
Larissa Pryor

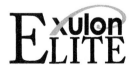

To Connie,

I hope you enjoy this true story
of a little boy who overcame
challenges + grew up to become Papa.

Amanda Graves
Dan "Papa" Graves

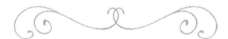

For Ben

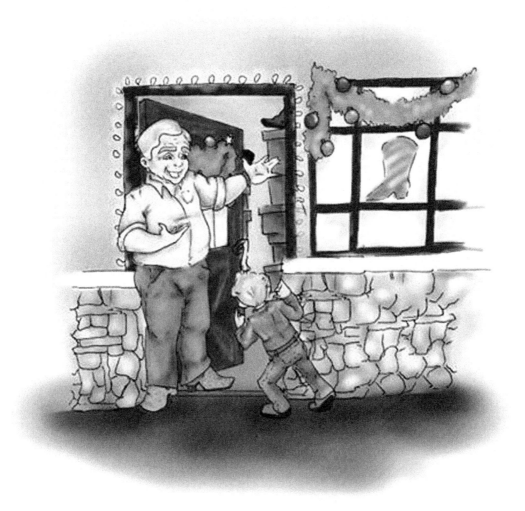

It was a chilly day just before Christmas when Papa took Jack to buy his first pair of cowboy boots.

There were rows and rows and rows of boots in the children's section. They were stacked from the floor as high as Papa's head. It was hard to know where to start.

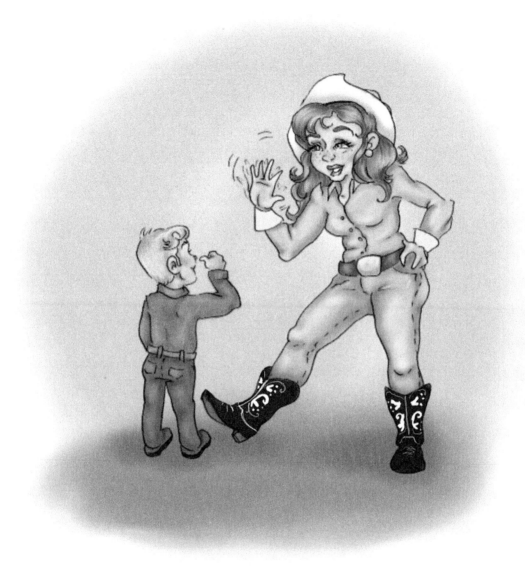

A lady in a cowboy hat came over to help them. Her boots were fancy.
"Howdy! My name's Sam," she said with a smile. "Who's buying boots today?"
"Me!" shouted Jack. "Papa's buying me my first pair!"
He tugged on Papa's hand and pointed to a pair of boots with a Texas star. "Can I try those?"

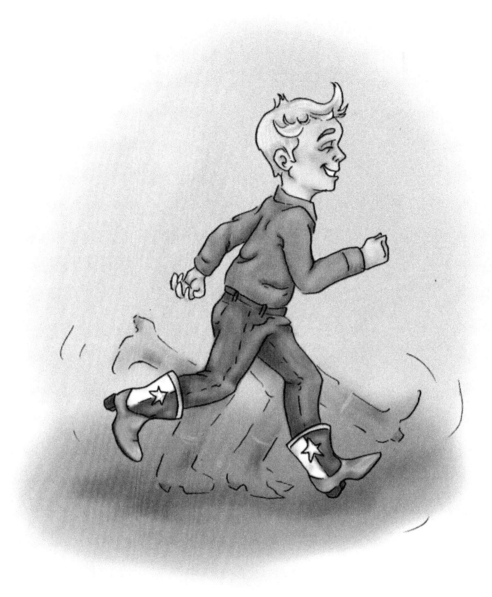

Sam found Jack's size and fetched them down. Jack wriggled and stomped with excitement as Sam helped him pull them on. As soon as his toes were all the way in, he took off running to see how they felt.

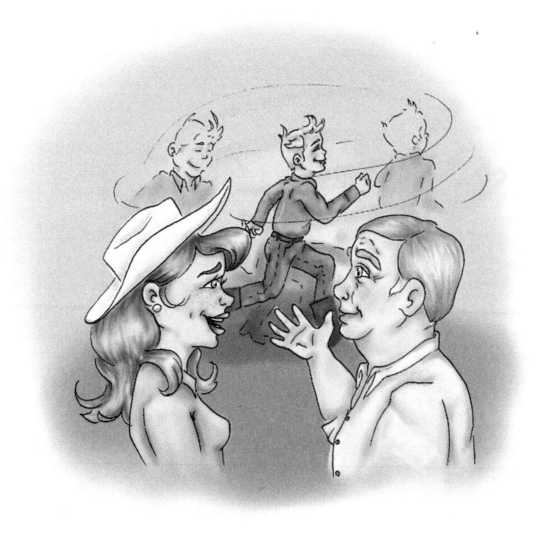

"How about you, sir?" asked Sam. "Are you planning on buying a pair today as well?"
There was a pause while Papa watched Jack run around the store.
"Not today," said Papa softly. "Today is just for my grandson. I want him to try on as many boots as he wants, run around, get excited and pick out the perfect pair. This could take a while."

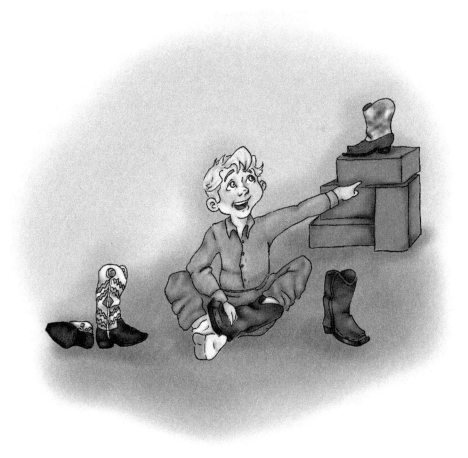

Jack came racing back.

"Can I try on those boots too?" he asked, bouncing up and down and pointing at a camou-flage pair. He was already pulling off the boots he was wearing.

"Sure!" said Sam. She found them in his size but this time he pulled them on all by himself. Then he took off running again.

This happened seven more times, and each pair was more handsome than the last.

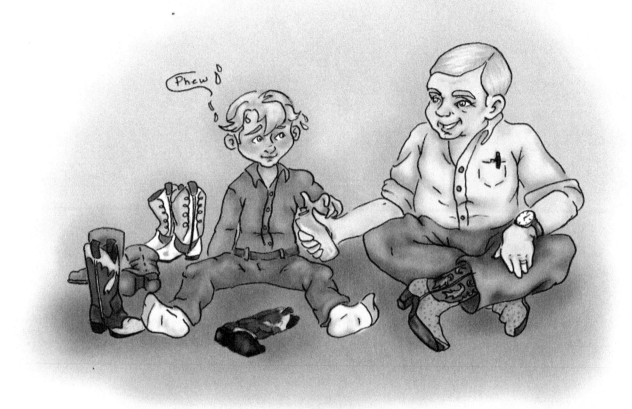

Finally, Jack was tired. Boots lay all over the floor. He sat down in the middle of them and Papa gave him a water bottle.

Papa gingerly lowered himself to the floor and sat down next to Jack.

"Shall I tell you about my first pair of cowboy boots?" he asked.

"OK," said Jack, and he lay down with his head on an empty box. Sam started picking up the scattered boots and trying to match them with their mates.

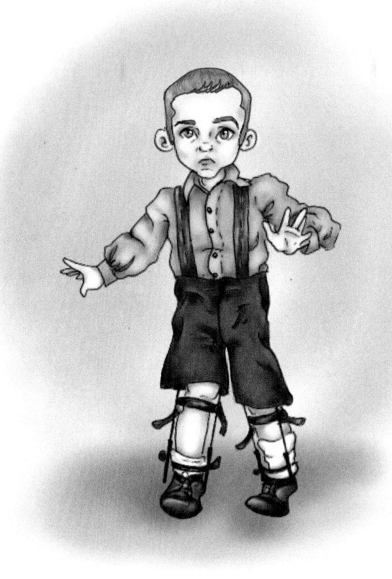

"Until I was just about your age," began Papa, "I wore braces on my legs."
"What's braces?" asked Jack.
"I don't guess you've ever seen anything like them, Jack," said Papa. "They were made from heavy straps which kept my legs straight below the knee. I couldn't run like the other kids, or play sports. I got real good at throwing a baseball, though!"

12

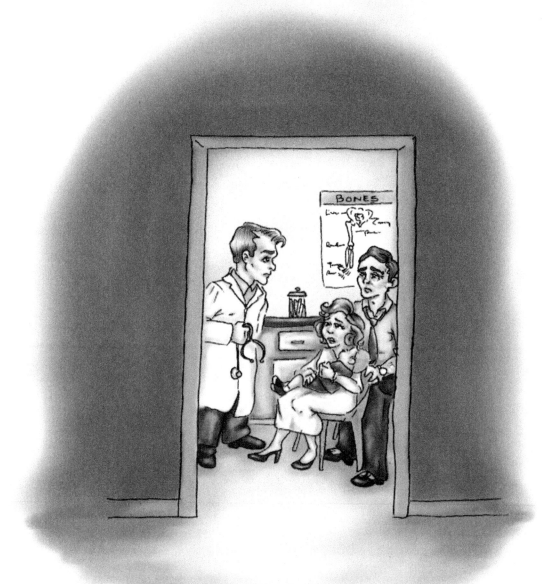

"But why did you have to wear braces?" asked Jack, frowning.

"One day when I was two years old," said Papa, "I woke up with a high fever and couldn't move at all. Not my arms or my legs. You know what it's like when your foot goes to sleep? Well, my whole body felt like that. My mom and dad rushed me to the hospital. I was real sick with a disease called polio. The doctors said I might never walk again. Lots of kids with polio never got better. I was lucky. I did. But I needed braces because my legs were pretty weak."

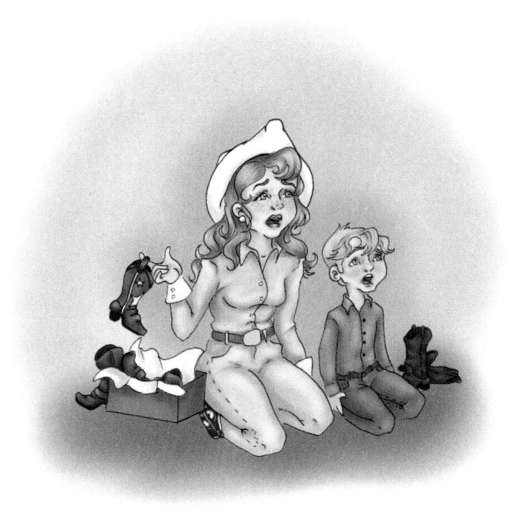

Now both Jack and Sam were staring at Papa. Sam was frozen, holding one boot on the end of her finger.

"How long did you have to wear the braces?" she asked.

"Four years," said Papa. "I didn't get them taken off until I was in first grade."

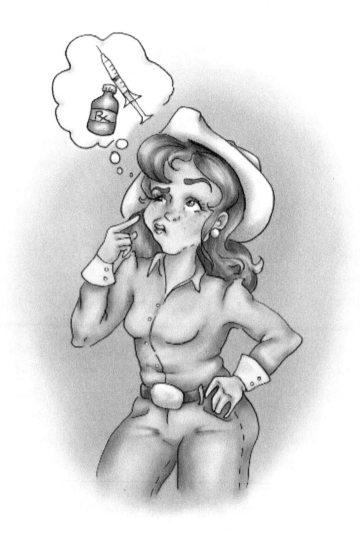

Sam looked puzzled.

"I've never heard of polio," she said.

"That's because nobody gets it any more," said Papa. "I was one of the last people in America to have it before a doctor came up with a vaccine to stop it. When you were a baby, Sam - and you too, Jack - you got that vaccine so you would never catch it. But sometimes you might see an older lady or gentleman using a wheelchair or a walker, and they might have had polio when they were little. Not everybody got all the way better.

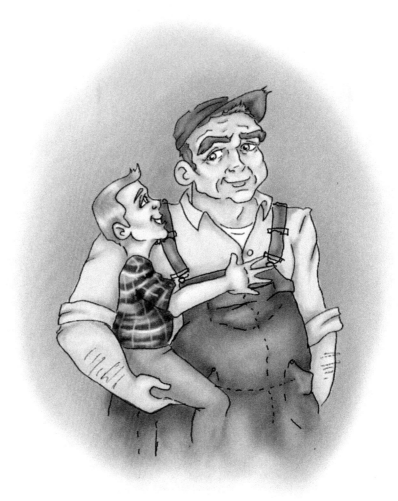

"When I turned six and the braces came off, boy did I want a pair of cowboy boots. My mother and father just couldn't afford them, though. My daddy was a small-town preacher who didn't get paid much, so my own Papa took me to buy my first pair. Everyone in town knew him; they called him Big H. He took me into the dry goods store and told everyone that this was a special day, and to make sure his grandson got the best pair they had. Now this wasn't a big store like where we are now. It was a little bitty place so we didn't have much to choose from. But that didn't matter. I know you're excited today, but can you imagine how excited I was? I was ten times happier than you are because I had never even worn a pair of regular shoes. So to pick out a pair of boots made me the happiest boy in town, maybe in the whole world."

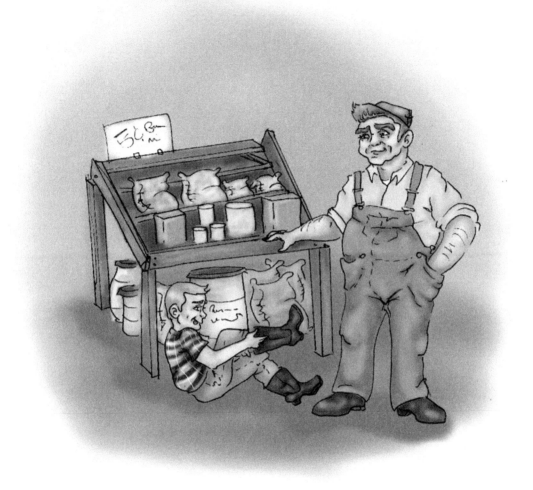

"What did they look like?" asked Jack.

"Well, Jack, I don't recall - but I probably have a photo somewhere. I just remember how happy I was that Big H. took me to buy them," said Papa. "He was a tough old guy. I never remember him reading me a story or putting me to bed or anything like that, but I guess he knew that this was the most important thing he could ever do for me."

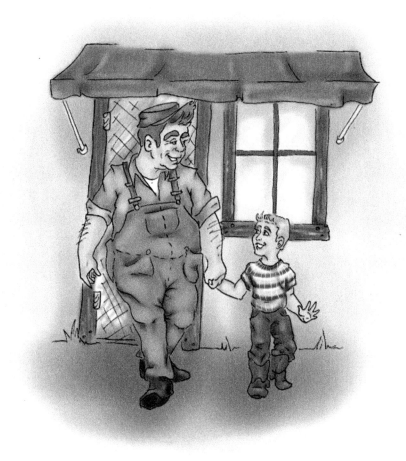

Papa stood up slowly, and Jack jumped to his feet.

"Where's Big H. now? Can I meet him?"

Papa turned away for a second.

"Next time you come to my house, I'll try to find that picture," he said. "Wouldn't that be cool?"

"Yeah!" said Jack.

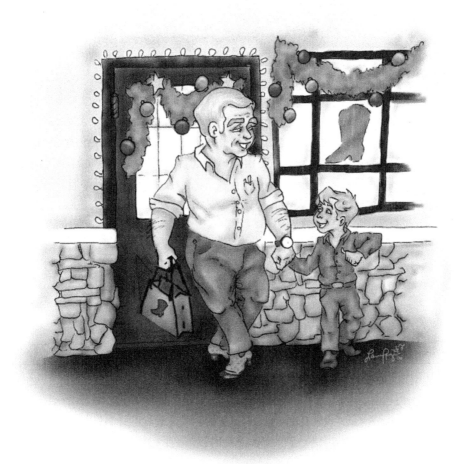

By now, Sam had all the boots lined up in a row.

"Before I put any of them back into their boxes, Jack," she said, "have you decided which pair you would like?"

Jack looked down at all the boots, thought for a moment, then smiled.

"I'm going to let Papa choose," he said.

About the author

Amanda Graves was born and educated in England and moved to the USA in 1985. She was a children's bookseller for five years while raising her own children, before opening a catering business. She currently divides her time between her extended blended family in Texas and Massachusetts, where she volunteers with at-risk students by teaching healthy eating classes in inner-city schools. Her husband Ben, a polio survivor, is the inspiration for "Papa's Boots."

About the illustrator

Larissa Pryor resides in San Antonio, Texas and is a clinical application analyst for a hospital corporation. She is the mother of five year old Oliver and three year old Ophelia. She studied to be an illustrator and aspires to own her own art studio. She is excited to join the author on her journey to achieve the vision of "Papa's Boots."

CPSIA information can be obtained
at www.ICGtesting.com
Printed in the USA
BVOW10s0543270816
460125BV00003B/3/P